FACTS
ON
FAD DIETS

Trendy Dietary Pattern Known To Be A
Quick Fix For Long Term Problems

VIENNA ROFFE

DISCLAIMER NOTE
This book is only intended to provide knowledge that is relevant to daily life.
Every effort has been made to provide accurate, current, trustworthy, and comprehensive information. In any way should you take this as medical advice; instead, you should speak with your physician.

TABLE OF CONTENT

INTRODUCTION

Successful weight loss is losing weight and keeping it off for at least 5 years. This can be achieved by making positive changes to both eating habits and physical activity. Fad diets won't work in long-term weight loss because the practices don't promote healthy and sustainable diets.

 These are the tactics that this book will concentrate on.

Food-specific fad diets depend on the myth that some foods have special parcels that can result in weight loss or gain but no food can. These diets do not educate healthy eating habits; thus, you will not stick with them for very long. Sooner or after, you will return to your normal eating habits and gain back all(if not further) of the weight you lost while on a fad diet.

By the end of this book, you'll have an in-depth knowledge of effective ways without having to do some ridiculous things.

Enjoy your read

SECTION 1

INSUFFICIENT PHYSICAL ACTIVITY

The health benefits of physical activity are nicely set up and consist of a lower hazard of cardiovascular disease, hypertension, diabetes, and breast and colon cancers. Additionally, bodily activity has tremendous effects on intellectual health, delays the onset of dementia, and may assist in the maintenance of a healthy weight.

Insufficient bodily pastime is a leading chance issue for non-communicable illnesses and has a negative impact on intellectual fitness and exceptional existence.

The Harmful Effects That Will Occur Due To Insufficient Physical Activity
Heart Disease

Not getting enough bodily activity can cause coronary heart disease even for human beings who've no different chance elements. It also can boost the chance of growing different heart disorder danger elements, inclusive of weight problems, excessive blood pressure, high blood cholesterol, and type 2 diabetes.

Type 2 Diabetes

Not getting sufficient physical pastime can increase a person's chance of developing kind 2 diabetes. Physical pastime enables the manipulation of blood sugar (glucose), weight, and blood pressure and "desirable" cholesterol and lower "awful" cholesterol. Adequate bodily activity at least one hundred fifty minutes of mild activity a week also can assist lessen the threat of coronary heart disorder and nerve harm, which might be regular troubles for human beings with diabetes.

Cancer

Getting the advocated quantity of bodily activity can lower the danger of many cancers, including cancers of the breast, colon, and uterus. Regular bodily interest is one of the most crucial matters human beings can do to improve their health. Moving more and sitting less have first-rate advantages for anyone, no matter age, sex, race, ethnicity, or current health stage.

Lack of physical activity has truly been proven to be a chance aspect for cardiovascular sickness and different conditions:

Less active and less matched people have more danger of growing excessive blood stress.

Physical activity can lessen your chance of type 2 diabetes.

Studies show that physically energetic humans are less likely to broaden coronary heart disease than inactive people. Lack of physical activity can upload to emotions of hysteria and despair.

Physical inaction may additionally boost the chance of sure cancers.

Physically active obese or obese human beings considerably reduced their risk for disease with everyday bodily activity.

Older adults who are physically energetic can lessen their threat of falls and improve their potential to do everyday sports.

Facts About Inactive Life

Thousands and heaps of deaths occur every year due to a loss of everyday bodily interest. In addition:

Inactivity has a tendency to grow with age.

Women are more likely to guide inactive life than men.

Non-Hispanic white adults are more likely to engage in physical interest than Hispanic and black adults.

Negative Effects of Inactivity

Physical activity, anything from doing chores to going for walks, is key to enhancing health. But what takes place in your body while it's sedentary?

Health Risks of Inactivity

According to The Department of Health and Human Services, eighty% of all Americans are not meeting current bodily pastime recommendations. They say this contributes to numerous persistent fitness conditions and that physical pastime, specifically moderate-to-energetic activity, can help offset these risks.

Short Term Effects

Any individuals who lead an inactive lifestyle position themselves with a greater chance of:

Anxiety
Depression
Weight Gain
Weakened immune system
Hormonal imbalance
Poor blood movement
A lower in skeletal muscular tissues
High levels of cholesterol

Long Term Effects

Lack of inaction also has long term consequences.
Over time, a sedentary way of life can result in extra
critical fitness conditions which include:

Coronary Heart Disease
Stroke
Type-2 Diabetes
Certain cancers which can result in death.

SECTION 2

UNINTENDED WEIGHT LOSS

Unintended weight loss is when you shed pounds
without converting your food plan or workout
habitually. It may be a sign of strain or a severe
infection.
It might be due to a traumatic event like a divorce,
dropping a task, or the demise of a loved one. It also
can be because of malnutrition, a health situation, or
an aggregate of factors,
intellectual fitness situations, which include
melancholy, anxiety, eating disorders, and
obsessive-compulsive disease (OCD)

troubles with digestion, including coeliac disorder or irritable bowel syndrome (IBS), different health situations, inclusive of an overactive thyroid, type 2 diabetes, or heart failure
Sometimes weight loss can be because of cancer. It's vital to get it checked in case you're dropping weight without trying.

Unintended weight loss can be due to situations that vary from moderate to very serious. The causes can be bodily or psychological, and encompass:

An overactive or underactive thyroid gland
The thyroid gland helps alter your body temperature and control your coronary heart price and metabolism (the technique that turns the meals you eat into electricity).

Addison's disorder
A situation in which the adrenal glands, which take a seat on top of the kidneys, do not produce enough of the hormones cortisol and aldosterone

Cancer
Crohn's sickness (an irritation of the bowels)
Parkinson's ailment

Heart failure

AIDS

Gastrointestinal troubles, together with peptic
ulcer or ulcerative colitis

Dental problems

Depression or anxiety

Side effects of prescription medicinal drugs

Celiac ailment (hypersensitivity to gluten)

Diabetes

A parasitic infection

Drug abuse

Undiagnosed consuming problems

Swelling of the pancreas

Alcohol or drug abuse

Dysphagia (swallowing issues)

Dementia.

SECTION 3

DETRIMENTAL FOR THOSE WITH CHRONIC ILLNESS

Chronic ailments remain long-term, regularly for 12 months or greater. You may also need ongoing hospital treatment and difficulties doing the belongings you want to do each day. These behaviors, known as activities of daily living, encompass such things as using the toilet and getting dressed. These difficulties also can affect your family. Examples of continual illnesses include diabetes and persistent lung sickness, along with COPD.

When you have an acute illness which includes bronchitis or the flu, you already know you'll feel higher and be lower back to ordinary inside a brief time frame. This isn't authentic with continual contamination. It may additionally by no means depart and may disrupt your lifestyles in some of the approaches.

Chronic illnesses have disorder-specific signs, however, may additionally bring invisible signs like aches, fatigue, and temper disorders. Pain and fatigue may also end up a frequent part of your day. Along with your infection, you probably have certain things you need to do to take care of yourself, like taking medication or doing sporting activities. Keeping up together with your fitness management tasks can also cause strain.

Physical adjustments from sickness may additionally affect your look. These changes can move an effective self-picture right into a terrible one. When you do not feel true about yourself, you may withdraw from pals and social activities. Mood disorders including melancholy and anxiety are commonplace proceedings of humans with persistent situations, however, they're extraordinarily treatable.

Chronic contamination can also affect your capacity to work. You would possibly exchange the way you work to deal with morning stiffness, decreased variety of motion, and different physical obstacles. If you aren't capable of painting, you might have financial problems.

If you're a homemaker, your paintings can also take much longer to do. You might want to ask for help from your spouse, a relative, or a home healthcare provider. As your lifestyle adjusts, you can feel a loss of management, anxiety, and uncertainty about your destiny. In some households, there might be a role reversal where folks that have been capable of staying at home must go back to painting.

Stress can build and may form your feelings about lifestyles. Long durations of strain can lead to frustration, anger, hopelessness, and, in some instances, depression. This can show up not handiest to you, but also to your family members. They're additionally inspired by using the chronic health issues of a cherished one.

These techniques permit you to regain the experience of managing and improving your fineness of life, something absolutely everyone deserves. If stricken by depression, your provider may prescribe medications to help adjust your mood and make you sense better.

There are, of the route, things that you could do for your very own with a purpose to assist. These include suggestions:

1. Eating a healthy weight loss plan.
2. Get as good a bodily activity as you can.
3. Avoiding bad coping mechanisms like alcohol and substance abuse.
4. Exploring strain-alleviation activities like meditation.

5. Letting off responsibilities that you don't
    need to do or want to do.
6. Asking for assistance whilst you want it.
7. Staying in contact with family and buddies.

SECTION 4

MAINTENANCE ISSUES

Deprivation

A calorie deficit promotes weight reduction. But
depriving yourself of the foods you enjoy to cut
calories is not the right thing to do.

And whilst fad diets may additionally help you shed
pounds in the short period, they're difficult to stick
to in the long run because of their restrictive nature.
It's also essential to take into account that body
weight is just one piece of the larger puzzle that
makes up a healthy person. Emerging studies
additionally show that weight may not have as big
an effect on health as specialists once believed.
If you're concerned about being wholesome, a
current look indicates that physical activity can be
greater critical than weight loss.

Of course, your eating regimen and body weight can impact fitness markers like blood stress and cholesterol, however, making weight reduction the stop-all-be-all aim might not be the first-rate method.

And relying on a short repair like a fad diet may motivate extra damage than proper.

CertainTrusted Source restrictive diets may also boost the chance of developing ingesting ailment tendencies in human beings of all sizes.

And even as a brief-restoration food regimen might enhance health markers in the brief term, until you're changing your habits for the lengthy haul, the upgrades, like better blood sugar management, may not be long-lasting.

Moreover, a restriction can result in cravings. Researchers are nonetheless looking to recognize meal cravings, but completely slicing out chocolate, potato chips, or ice cream can lead you to want one's meals more than ever. Deprivation isn't a possible lengthy-time period answer because it's not sustainable.

The restriction mindset can cause binging and similarly restrict a dangerous cycle that could cause weight-cycling, that's associated with a better threat of ailment and mortality.

There's additionally a capability associationTrusted Source among restrictive weight-reduction plans and the improvement of ingesting problems.

Removing your favorite meals additionally takes away lots of delight in eating. It's viable to revel in the ingredients you love and nevertheless attain your fitness desires.

One of the main tenets of Intuitive Eating, as an example, is mild nutrition, the idea that you can eat healthfully whilst honoring your taste buds.

Nutrient deficiencies

Often, certain ingredients or macronutrients become the target of fad diets. But in case you're required to cut out a whole meals organization, the eating regimen likely gained at closing. You will also be at a higher chance of nutrient deficiencies.

Cutting out foods and meal corporations, or extensively lowering caloric intake, could make it tougher to get the nutrients your frame wishes.

For example, human beings following a strict vegan eating regimen are at riskTrusted Source for nutrition B12 deficiency because the nutrient is found on the whole in animal foods.

And in case you devour a completely low-carb weight loss program, like the keto food plan, you can now not be getting enough trusted Source fiber or different key nutrients and minerals, which can lead to unsightly side effects like constipation and muscle cramps.

Unnecessarily demonizing positive foods

Your weight loss plan doesn't want to involve an all-or-nothing technique. Some ingredients are extra nutritious than others, however, all meals may be a part of a wholesome weight loss program. We live in an international of delicious alternatives, in any case.

Of course, too much of a tasty aspect may negatively impact your fitness. Large quantities of delicate carbs, for an instance, can cause trusted Source blood sugar spikes that could ultimately lead to trusted Source diabetes. They can also contributeTrusted Source to the development of heart sickness. Carbs aren't the enemy, though. You can lessen your delicate carbs and sugar intake without going to the extreme. Whole grains, fruits, vegetables, and legumes comprise masses of nutrients, inclusive of fiber, that is critical for gut fitness.

Disordered eating

Diets also can negatively impact your intellectual fitness.

Fad diets, in particular, are related to trusted Sources a multiplied risk of disordered ingesting and eating disorders due to their restrictive nature and bad impact on the framed picture.

There's also the intellectual toll of restricting recall. Constantly striving to "devour flawlessly" can cause pointless pressure, which may, in turn, have an effect on your overall fitness.

Changes to attempt instead of fad diets

Are you trying to enhance your usual health? Here's what to try in preference to that famous fad weight loss program that's throughout your social media feeds.

Be regular

Eat continually in the day to help maintain ideal blood sugar degrees, save you indigestion, and scale back uncomfortable bloating.

Eat balanced food

Aim for your food to encompass lean protein, carbs high in fiber, and healthy fats. Not simplest will this help you consume a spread of nutrient-wealthy

meals, but, it'll additionally stabilize your blood
sugar and sell a healthy gut microbiota.

Focus on adding in preference to eliminating
Eat more culmination and vegetables! Aim for four–
5 servings daily. What's a serving? One cup of leafy
greens, 1/2 cup of cooked vegetables, a chunk of
fruit approximately the scale of a tennis ball, or
approximately 1 cup of berries. If that appears like
masses, begin slowly and add a serving to at least
one meal or snack. Remember that canned, frozen,
and dried produce matter quantity too, but try to
pick out ones and not use a little delivered sugar
and salt.

Be conscious of introduced sugar
It's a very good idea to maintain delivered sugar
intake as little as feasible for the simplest fitness.
You'll find out that sugar is brought in candy meals,
like cookies and ice cream, however, it's also in lots
of specific components like bread, crackers, and
yogurt. Added sugar shows up on food labels under
numerous names: honey, agave, inverted sugar,
sucrose, and fructose. Try to pick out lower sugar
options at the same time as you can.

Enjoy the food you like

Complete deprivation doesn't paint. If you're concerned about sugar intake, having a few desserts every night time can also help cut back extreme sweet cravings. Restrictive diets tell you in no way to have dessert, leading to cravings and binging. Because you inform yourself you'll in no way consume cookies over again, eating one cookie can change into eating an entire field. Allowing yourself to enjoy the food you adore without the guilt whether or not that's chocolate, ice cream, or cookies can genuinely be a part of a healthy food regimen.

Get transferring

You don't want to start doing excessive-intensity workouts at 5 am To improve your fitness. Getting at least 150 mins of mild- interest every week can extensively reduce your chance of coronary heart ailment and stroke. That's simply over 21 mins a day and may encompass any interest that receives your coronary heart charge up, which incorporates brisk walking and household chores.

Regular exercise is likewise proper for your bones and can help beautify your sleep greatly. Moving your frame can also have a notable impact on your intellectual health.

SECTION 5

SHORT TERMS CHANGES

These diets offer brief and painless weight reduction at the same time as allowing the consumption of preferred or tasty meals, however, place excessive restrictions on positive other elements or meal training. Fad diets regularly work within the short term because they'll be low-kilojoule diets in hiding; this is, strength consumption because the weight loss plan is lower than the character's necessities. Successful long-term weight loss is based upon consumption over an extended period of less electricity than is expended. The ideal approach is to boost bodily activity whilst enhancing consuming behavior to achieve a nutritionally balanced consumption.

A fad healthy eating plan is a weight loss program that turns into well-known for a short time, much like fads in style, without being a fashionable dietary recommendation, and regularly making pseudoscientific or unreasonable claims for instant weight loss or health upgrades. Diets are famous non-popular diets that frequently promise dramatic weight loss. However, they may be commonly not supported with the aid of clinical evidence, and they sometimes offer risky nutritional recommendations.

Generally, fad diets promise a series of short-time period changes requiring little to no attempt; attracting the pursuits of uneducated customers about complete-weight loss programs, and whole-manner of life changes critical for sustainable health benefices. Fad diets are regularly promoted with exaggerated claims, together with rapid weight loss of greater than 1 kg/week, enhancing health by way of using "cleaning", or perhaps volatile claims, inclusive of relatively restrictive and nutritionally unbalanced meals alternatives main to malnutrition or eating non-food gadgets like cotton wool. Highly restrictive fad diets want to be prevented. At exceptional, fad diets may additionally offer novel and attractive ways to lessen caloric consumption, however at worst they'll be medically wrong to the individual, unsustainable, or maybe volatile. Dietitian recommendations ought to be favored earlier than trying any diet plan. They generally tend to result in short-time period weight reduction, however afterward, the weight is often regained. The restrictive method, no matter whether or not or now not the diet prescribes consuming big amounts of immoderate-fiber vegetables, no grains, or no strong foods, has the propensity to be nutritionally unsound and may cause excessive fitness problems if found for days. A massive drawback of fad diets is they encourage the notion of an eating regimen as brief-time period conduct, in preference to a sustainable lifelong trade. Indeed, fad diets regularly fail to re-teach dieters approximately healthy vitamins, component control, and under-emphasize efforts in particular physical activity, so that fans can't collect the abilities and understanding they want for lengthy-time period maintenance in their preferred weight, even though that weight is finished inside the quick-time period.

Several diets are also unsustainable in the prolonged term, and as a result, dieters revert to antique conduct after deprivation of a few ingredients which may additionally lead to binge ingesting. Fad diets commonly fail to deal with the reasons for horrible nutrient conduct, and consequently are unlikely to exchange the underlying conduct and the prolonged-time period outcomes.

Some fad diets are related to increased risks of cardiovascular illnesses, kidney stones, and intellectual issues consisting of eating issues and despair, and dental dangers. For instance, prolonged-time period low-carbohydrate immoderate-fat diets are associated with prolonged cardiac and non-cardiac mortality. Teenagers following fad diets are prone to permanently stunted growth.

Some fad diets do but provide short-term and lengthy-term outcomes for human beings with specific ailments including obesity or epilepsy. Very-low-calorie diets, moreover referred to as crash diets, are green for liver fats bargain and weight reduction earlier than bariatric surgical remedy. Low-calorie and truly-low-calorie diets may also moreover produce, to begin with, faster weight loss within the first 1–2 weeks of starting in comparison to other diets, however, this superficially quicker loss is because of glycogen depletion and water loss in the lean frame mass and regained speedy later on.

Diet fulfillment in weight loss and health benefits is most expected via adherence and horrible electricity stability, regardless of the food plan type. Fad diets, with their popularity and variety, may be useful to introduce obese people thru a dietary plan tailor-made to their meals choices and lifestyle into long-time period dietary and way-of-life modifications beneath supervision by nutrition specialists. Indeed, a wide type of diets aiming at mild caloric restriction below supervision, which includes industrial, fad, and tremendous care diets, have shown extraordinary and comparable fulfillment and safety, every within a brief-time period and lengthy period. Comprehensive weight-loss program packages are more powerful than a weight-reduction plan without guidance. Efforts to beautify public health through weight-reduction plans are forestalled no longer for the need, knowledge approximately the pinnacle-rated feeding of Homo sapiens however for distractions associated with exaggerated claims, and our failure to convert what we reliably realize into what we robotically do.

SECTION 6

INSUFFICIENT NUTRIENTS

A weight loss plan that is done with the wrong approach continuously will result in insufficient nutrients. Inadequate nutrients can disrupt the metabolic procedures in the frame, one every of which is hypoglycemia. In Indonesia, there are few effective studies about eating conduct because it's far though considered a trivial trouble. In fact, this consuming disorder may be as a result of several incorrect perceptions, collectively with the notion that a thin frame is the satisfactory frame form, for that reason triggering ladies to make numerous efforts to shed kilos immediately because of the low mental factors and understanding elements. Inadequate nutrient intake in the frame, together with the result of fad food regimen, might probably increase the risk of health troubles in the end. Fad diets can affect dietary fame and nutritional insufficiency. Malnourished refers to not receiving enough of any of the essential factors of the weight-reduction plan: proteins, fat, carbohydrates, nutrients, minerals, and water. Insufficient portions of any of these can be just as dangerous as caloric malnourishment. Unfortunately, nutrient deficiencies and malnutrition can persist for a long term before they show up in physical signs and symptoms.

1. Unexplained Fatigue

Fatigue is a commonplace aspect effect of iron deficiency, which can cause anemia, indicated through low tiers of crimson blood cells. Anemia can also display bizarre paleness. But keep in thoughts: Other situations can cause excessive fatigue, which incorporates coronary heart sickness, despair, or thyroid sickness. It's clever to alert your health practitioner if you sense exceedingly vulnerability or worn out. Your medical doctor can also prescribe dietary supplements when you have anemia.

2. Brittle and Dry Hair

Hair, that's made up extra regularly than no longer of protein, serves as a beneficial diagnostic marker for dietary deficiencies.
Brittle hair can sign a deficit of essential fatty acids, protein, iron, and other vitamins. Some hair loss is normal with age. But if hair starts to fall out at an unusual charge, nutrient deficiencies may be the

purpose. Once your medical doctor identifies the deficiencies, you could treat them with nutrient-rich meals and dietary supplements.

3. Ridged or Spoon-Shaped Nails

Like hair, nails function as an early warning sign of an inadequate weight loss plan. A spoon-shaped nail, in which the nail curves up from the nail bed like a spoon (a situation referred to as koilonychia) may be a trademark of iron-deficiency anemia.
If you have iron-deficiency anemia, you may additionally advise iron capsules and iron-rich food which includes liver and shellfish like clams, oysters, and mussels.

4. Mouth Problems

Cracking or infection on the corners of the mouth (a situation referred to as angular cheilitis) may be a warning sign of both riboflavin (B2) deficiency or iron deficiency. A surprisingly mild or swollen tongue is a cautious sign of iron or B-vitamins deficiency. A state of affairs referred to as burning mouth syndrome, which continues to puzzle researchers, might also additionally get up while iron, zinc, or B-vitamins tiers fall below the specified stage. Again, as soon as you've confirmed your particular dietary deficiencies, they may be handled with nutrient-wealthy ingredients and nutritional supplements.

5. Diarrhea

Chronic diarrhea can be a signal of malabsorption, this means that nutrients are not being completely absorbed with the resource of your frame. Malabsorption can be brought approximately through infection, surgical treatment, certain capsules, heavy alcohol use, and digestive troubles which include celiac sprue and Crohn's ailment. It's critical to seek advice from your clinical physician if you have continual diarrhea.

6. Apathy or Irritability

Unexplained temper modifications, especially feeling apathetic or irritable, may be signs and signs of a severe medical circumstance like depression. But they also can be signs and signs that your frame isn't getting the power it dreams. If you have a persistent low temper or forgetfulness, it's vital to get checked

7. Lack of Appetite

With age, the urge for meals regularly diminishes. Taste buds lose their sensitivity. If you furthermore might become tons less energetic, you might also need less energy. Medications also can hose down the urge for meals.

A Chronic lack of urge for food is an extreme caution sign that you may be susceptible to nutritional deficiencies. If you find yourself skipping food due to the reality you're not hungry, communicate with your loved ones.

Blood exams can mean in case you're deficient in some key vitamins. By assessing your meal consumption, a registered dietitian can also spot dietary deficiencies.

The vital issue is to alert your scientific medical doctor fast in case your urge for food modifications in any other case you begin skipping meals. In that manner, you could head off dietary problems in advance than they reason intense trouble.

SECTION 7

MISSING HEALTHY FOOD

Here are **12** of the healthiest non-perishable foods.

1. Dried and canned beans

With an extended shelf lifestyle and excessive nutrient content, dried and canned beans are clever non-perishable food alternatives. Canned beans may be saved at room temperature for 2–5 years whilst dried beans can last 10 or more years and counting. In truth, one has taken a look at discovering that pinto beans stored for as much as 30 years had been taken into consideration fit for human intake through 80% of human beings on an emergency meal.

Beans are an excellent supply of fiber, plant-based absolute protein, magnesium, B nutrients, manganese, iron, phosphorus, zinc, and copper. What's greater, they pair well with maximum meals and make hearty additions to soups, grain dishes, and salads.

2. Nut butter

Nut butter is creamy, nutrient-dense, and scrumptious.

Although garage temperatures will affect shelf life, business peanut butter keeps for as much as 9 months at room temperature. Natural peanut butter, which no longer comprises preservatives, lasts up to a few months at 50°F (10°C) and best 1 month at 77°F (25°C).

Nut butter is a rich source of healthy fat, protein, nutrients, minerals, and powerful plant compounds, together with phenolic antioxidants, which can be compounds that protect your frame from oxidative pressure and damage through volatile molecules called free radicals.

Jars of nut butter can be stored in your pantry whilst smaller packets can be taken backpacking or camping for an on-the-go snack.

3. Dried give up result and greens

Although most smooth cease results and greens have a quick shelf existence, dried produce is taken into consideration as non-perishable. When properly stored, most dried fruit can be correctly saved at room temperature for up to at least one year, and dried greens can be kept for about half of that time (8, 9, 10).

You can pick from an expansion of dried culmination and veggies, which includes dried

berries, apples, tomatoes, and carrots. You can also use a dehydrator or oven to make your very own dried fruits and vegetables. Vacuum-sealed packaging can help save you from spoilage.
Dried fruits and vegetables may be loved as a snack or brought to path combination. Plus, dried vegetables can be rehydrated with the aid of such as soups or stews if glowing produce isn't available.

4. Canned fish and chicken

Although sparkling fish and hen are full of nutrients, they're noticeably perishable. All the same, canned sorts can be successfully saved without refrigeration for lengthy intervals as an awful lot as five years at room temperature.

Tuna and distinct seafood products are also bought in lightweight applications known as retort pouches, which can be perfect for smaller pantries and backpacking. Seafood in retort pouches has a shelf life of as much as 18 months.

Chicken and exceptional meats may be discovered in retort pouches as nicely.

5. Nuts and seeds

Nuts and seeds are transportable, nutrient-dense, and shelf-strong, making them non-perishable meal staples. Favored by backpackers and hikers for high-calorie snacking, they're additionally tremendous to have reachable in any scenario.

On commonplace, nuts final approximately 4 months whilst kept at or near room temperature (68°F or 20°C), although shelf existence varies considerably among nut types.
For instance, cashews may be stored for 6 months at 68°F (20°C) while pistachios are most effective ultimate 1 month at an identical temperature.
Seeds have comparable shelf lives. Pumpkin seeds live clean for 6 months at room temperature.

6. Grains

Whole grains like oats, rice, and barely have a far longer shelf life than unique famous but perishable carb assets like bread, making them a clever desire for lengthy-time period food garages.
For instance, brown rice may be stored at 50–70°F (10–21°C) for up to a few months whilst farro lasts up to six months at room temperature.
Grains can be brought to soups, salads, and casseroles, making them a bendy non-perishable element. Plus, ingesting whole grains may also

lessen your danger of type 2 diabetes, coronary heart
disorder, and high-quality cancers.

7. Canned greens and give up the result
Canning has been used to extend the shelf existence
of perishable substances, which consist of the result
and greens.
The heat used during canning kills probably
dangerous microorganisms, and the functional seal
of canned foods maintains new microorganisms
from spoiling the contents.

The shelf existence of canned results and veggies
depends on the shape of the produce.

For example, low-acid canned veggies, together
with potatoes, carrots, beets, and spinach, close to
2–5 years at room temperature.

On the other hand, high-acid stop results like
grapefruit, apples, peaches, berries, and pineapple
very last truly 12–18 months. The equal is going for
vegetables packed in vinegar, collectively with
sauerkraut, German potato salad, and other pickled
vegetables.

When shopping, select out canned culmination packed in water or 100% fruit juice rather than heavy syrup and choose low sodium canned greens each time feasible.

If you're foxy within the kitchen, bear in mind canning at home the usage of store-provided or lawn-grown veggies and fruits.

8. Jerky

Meat safety is an exercise used in given historic times to hold protein resources from spoiling. Specifically, jerky is made by curing meat in a salt answer, then dehydrating it. Preservatives, flavorings, and other components are once in a while used in the course of processing. Many styles of jerky are available, which include red meat, salmon, bird, and buffalo. There are even plant-based jerky alternatives crafted from coconut, banana, and jackfruit. That said, a word that the alternatives are not nutritionally identical to meat-based jerkies. Any form of jerky may be loved carefully, however, the healthiest options are folks that don't compromise brought sugar, synthetic flavors, or preservatives.

9. Granola and protein bars

Granola and protein bars are a move to food for backpackers and hikers due to their prolonged shelf life and nutrient composition.

Many granola bars stay clean for up to at least 1 year at room temperature. Likewise, maximum protein bars have a shelf existence of at least 1 year, even though it's first-class to check the label on character merchandise for expiration date.

What's greater, granola and protein bars may be notably nutritious so long as you pick the right sorts. Look for manufacturers which can be whole of hearty elements, which include oats, nuts, and dried fruit, and include minimal introduced sugars and synthetic components.

10. Soup

Canned and dried soups are a great desire when stocking your pantry. They're additionally desired by way of meal donation organizations. Most canned soups are low in acid and might last as long as 5 years at room temperature. The exception is tomato-primarily based kinds, which have a shelf life of approximately 18 months.

Although most dried soup mixes ought to last as long as 1year in storage, it's notable to test labels for expiration dates. Choose soups that are probably wealthy in healthful substances like veggies and beans, and choose low sodium merchandise on every occasion viable, as eating too much-added salt can also increase temperature.

11. Freeze-dried meals

Freeze drying uses sublimation, a procedure wherein ice is converted right away into vapor, to do away with water from meals simply so it lasts longer at room temperature. Freeze-dried meals are well-known amongst backpackers due to their mild weight and portability.

Freeze-dried elements and equipped to devour freeze-dried food are made for a prolonged-time period garage with a few products boasting a 30-year taste guarantee.

12. Shelf-robust milk and nondairy milk

While easy milk and some non dairy alternatives like almond and coconut milk ought to be refrigerated, shelf-solid milk and masses of non dairy milk are made to preserve at room temperature.

Shelf-strong or aseptic milk is processed and packaged in any other case than everyday milk as it's heated to higher temperatures and packed in sterile bins.

Shelf-stable milk had a shelf life of as much as nine months while saved at 40–68°F (4–20°C).

Plant-based liquids like soy milk packaged in flexible substances, collectively with plastic, paper, and aluminum, similarly last as long as 10 months, at the same time as canned coconut milk keeps as much as 5 years at room temperature

Shelf-solid and plant-based milk may be used while refrigeration isn't available. Powdered milk is a great opportunity, with a predicted shelf life of 3–5 years when saved in a cool, darkish area. It may be reconstituted with clean water in small quantities as wanted.

NOTE

Non-perishable ingredients last a long term without spoiling and are essential for numerous situations. Whether you need to donate items to charitable businesses, Them together for potential emergencies, buy backpacking-friendly merchandise, or simply inventory your pantry, you can pick out from an abundance of healthful elements that don't require refrigeration.